# Complete Acid-Reflux Cookbook for Beginners

## Relief from GERD with A 3-week Meal Plan, healthy and fast recipes

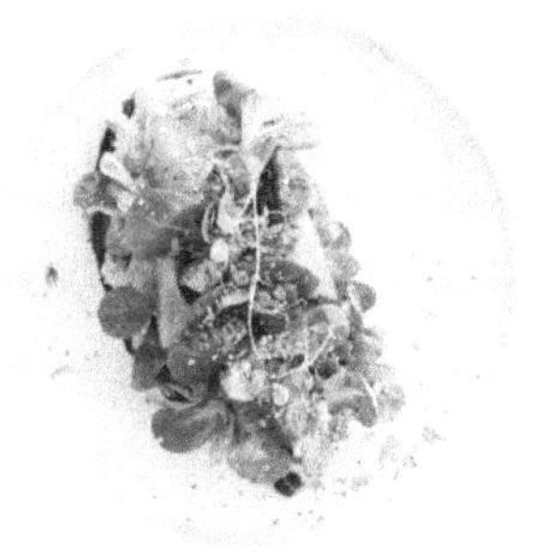

# Belinda Ross

*Complete Acid-Reflux Cookbook
for Beginners*

# Table Of Contents





*Complete Acid-Reflux Cookbook
for Beginners*

# Introduction

There was this amazing woman called Maria once upon a time. She sometimes had bad days due to the condition called acid reflux.

Maria never gave up! She decided to take control of the situation and put an end to her acid reflux.

Maria began by doing some internet research, but she avoided being confused by the complex medical terminology.

She discovered easy methods to relieve the symptoms of acid reflux.


*Complete Acid-Reflux Cookbook for Beginners*

She was all about keeping things simple and useful.

Maria started by altering her diet. She said farewell to the spiciness of the tacos and the cheese of the pizza and said welcome to the calming meals of yoghourt, oats, and bananas. Yum!

She discovered that eating smaller quantities also aided in preventing overeating.

Maria, however, was a cat with an inquisitive nature, so she continued.

She discovered that certain beverages might aggravate acid reflux. No more drinking acidic juices or fizzy drinks for her! She drank water and calming herbal drinks instead. Ah, how revitalising!

However, there's still more! Maria's focus extended beyond healthy eating. She was aware that stress may contribute to her acid reflux dance.

She thus incorporated some calming hobbies, like yoga and deep breathing, into her day. Her body and mind experienced it as a mini-vacation.

What about bedtime? That was also a major one! Before falling asleep, Maria said farewell to hefty dinners and late-night munchies.

To prevent the acid from rising at night, she slightly elevated the head of her bed. clever cookie, huh?

Maria also found several all-natural treatments that had miraculous results. Her stomach felt much better with a tablespoon of honey before night and some soothing aloe vera juice after meals.

7
*Complete Acid-Reflux Cookbook
for Beginners*

It resembled her special potion.

Maria's symptoms of acid reflux began to lessen. She felt better than ever before! No more unpleasant shocks that make her day miserable.

She was able to eat and enjoy life without those bothersome symptoms interfering.

You are not alone if you have experienced the misery of acid reflux.

Millions of people struggle with the effects of GERD, looking for solutions to reduce symptoms and live pain-free lives.

You and other novices who are ready to take control of their health and well-being are the target audience for this cookbook.

You will go on a gastronomic trip that transcends boring and constricting diets inside these pages.

Instead, we'll delve into a world of savoury, nutritious foods that have been skillfully created to ease acid reflux and savour your palate.

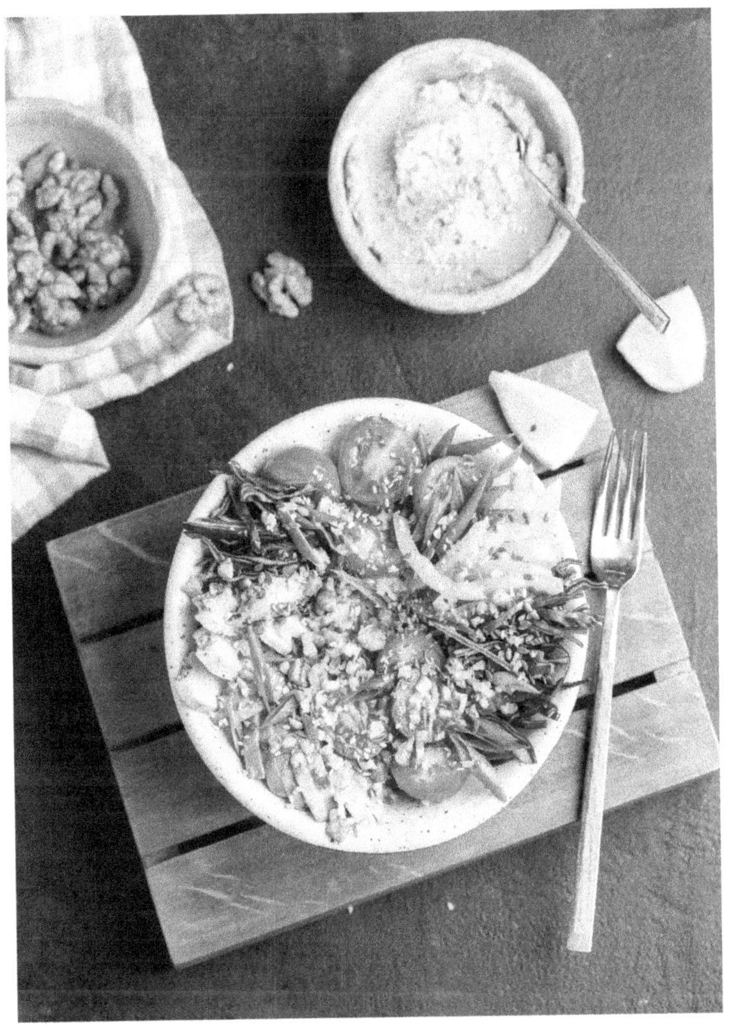

**10**
*Complete Acid-Reflux Cookbook
for Beginners*

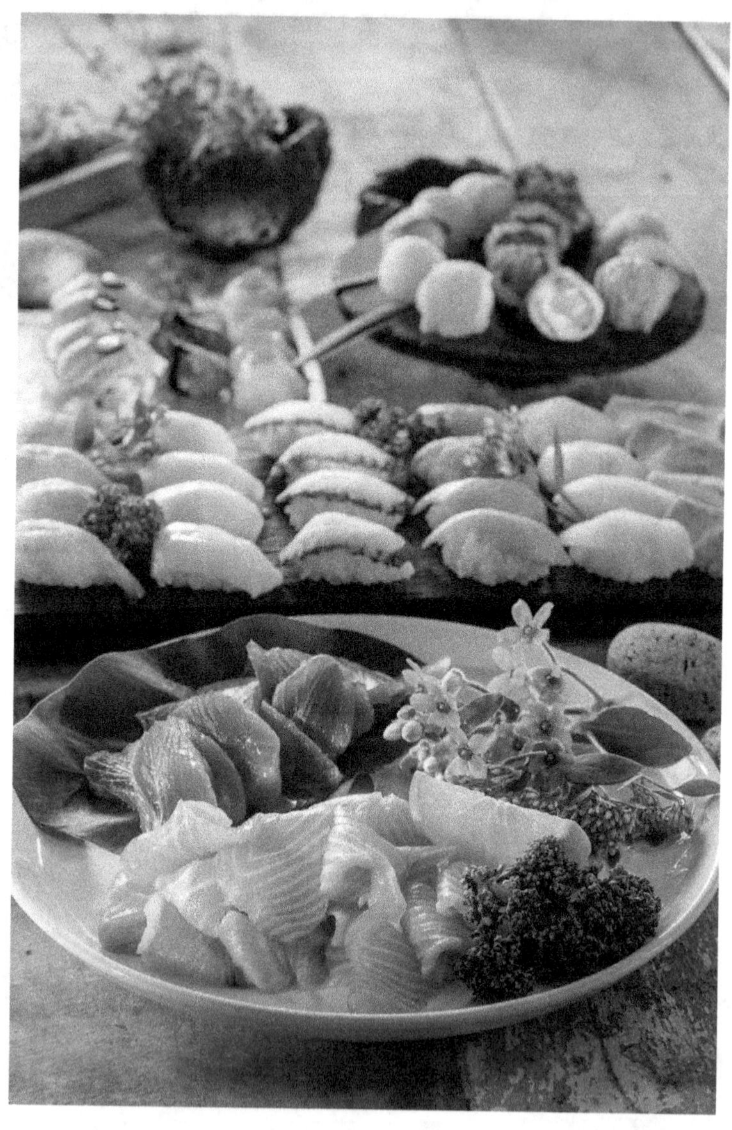

**11**
*Complete Acid-Reflux Cookbook
for Beginners*

# Chapter One

## Essential Elements of a GERD-Relief Diet

A cautious and conscientious approach to meal selections is necessary while living with GERD.

Particularly for people who have acid reflux, what we eat immediately affects how we feel.

The crucial elements of a GERD-relief diet will be covered in this chapter, with an emphasis on nutritious foods and critical nutrients that support digestive comfort and general well-being.

## What To Eat

**Lean Proteins:** Choose lean protein sources including skinless fish, chicken, and tofu.

These proteins provide crucial amino acids for muscle repair and general health and are less prone to cause acid reflux symptoms.

**Non-Citrus Fruits:** Apples, bananas, and melons are soft on the stomach and rich in vitamins and antioxidants, but citrus fruits may aggravate acid reflux.

**Whole Grains:** Include whole grains in your meals, such as brown rice, quinoa, and oats.

These grains help to support good digestion and lower the risk of heartburn while being high in fibre.

**Leafy Greens**: Leafy greens, especially dark leafy greens like Swiss chard, spinach, and kale, are a great source of vitamins, minerals, and antioxidants that help to maintain a healthy gut.

Sweet potatoes, carrots, and beets are mild on the stomach and provide important minerals including fibre and vitamin A.

Choose heart-healthy fats from foods like avocados, almonds, and olive oil. These fats may promote a healthy digestive tract and lower inflammation.

**Low-Fat Dairy:** Instead of full-fat dairy, which in some people may cause symptoms of acid reflux, choose low-fat or non-dairy substitutes such as almond milk or coconut milk.

**Herbs and spices:** To enhance taste and aid digestion, add mild herbs and spices like basil, ginger, and turmeric to your meals.

# What to Avoid

Knowledge is power when it comes to treating GERD and getting relief from acid reflux.

Understanding the foods and lifestyle choices that might exacerbate acid reflux symptoms is one of the


*Complete Acid-Reflux Cookbook
for Beginners*

essential components of a healthy GERD-friendly lifestyle.

You may make wise decisions and be proactive in easing discomfort and promoting digestive comfort by knowing what these triggers are.

## Foods That Aggravate the symptoms of Acid Reflux

Certain foods have a history of exacerbating acid reflux symptoms and serving as catalysts for pain.

Knowing these factors gives you the ability to avoid possible problems and choose things that are better for your digestive health.

Typical meals to stay away from include:

**Citrus Fruits:** Tomatoes, oranges, grapefruits, and lemons are all quite acidic and may cause heartburn.

**Spicy Foods:** Hot peppers, chilli, and other spicy foods may aggravate acid reflux symptoms by irritating the esophagus.

**Fatty and Fried meals:** High-fat meals, such as fried dishes, fatty meat cuts, and rich sweets, may cause acid reflux by slowing down digestion.

The lower esophageal sphincter may be loosened by mint and peppermint, enabling stomach acid to travel back up the esophagus.

**Carbonated Drinks:** Carbonated beverages, such as soda and sparkling water, may raise stomach pressure and cause acid reflux.

**Caffeinated Beverages:** Energy drinks, coffee, and tea may all relax the lower esophageal sphincter, which can lead to acid reflux.

**Garlic and onions:** For some people, these foods might cause heartburn and gastrointestinal distress.

**Chocolate:** This tasty indulgence may cause acid reflux by loosening the esophageal sphincter.

**Alcohol:** Beer, wine, and spirits may make acid reflux worse by causing the stomach to produce more acid.

**Foods Made of Tomatoes:** Some individuals may get symptoms while


*Complete Acid-Reflux Cookbook for Beginners*

eating acidic tomato sauces and pastes.

## Best Lifestyle Practices for GERD Relief

A few lifestyle choices may significantly contribute to GERD alleviation and general digestive comfort in addition to avoiding trigger foods.

You may assist your efforts to properly control acid reflux by adding these routines into your everyday life:

**Portion Control:** Eating too much may strain the stomach and make acid reflux more likely. Aim for more frequent, smaller meals.

**Maintain a Healthy Weight:** Focus on obtaining and keeping a healthy weight since excess weight might exacerbate GERD symptoms.

**Elevate Your Head**: By raising the head of your bed by six to eight inches as you sleep, you may lessen the risk of esophageal reflux disease.

**Keep Your Head Up After Eating**: Avoid reclining down soon away after eating as this might promote acid reflux. After eating, spend at least 2 to 3 hours doing light exercise or sitting up straight.

**Avoid Wearing Tight Clothes:** Wearing clothes that are too tight around the waist might cause strain on the stomach, which could lead to acid reflux.

**Quit Smoking:** Smoking may exacerbate the symptoms of acid reflux and weaken the lower esophageal sphincter.

**Manage Stress:** Use relaxation methods like deep breathing, meditation, or yoga to reduce stress, which may make GERD symptoms worse.

# Chapter Two

## 3-Week Meal Plan

Welcome to the first of your three-week journey to reduce acid reflux and adopt a GERD-friendly way of life.

You'll discover a carefully selected meal plan on these pages that is intended to help your digestive comfort and general well-being.

Your GERD relief journey will be fun and hassle-free thanks to the abundance of delectable, healthy, and simple-to-prepare foods on each day's menu.

## Week 1

### Day 1

**Breakfast:** banana walnut muffins.

**Lunch:** Chicken noodle soup for lunch

**Dinner:** Sauteed vegetables and cashew chicken

### Day 2

**Breakfast:** Buttermilk Pancakes with Fresh Berries for breakfast

**Lunch:** Eggplant soup for lunch

**Dinner:** Chicken with Quinoa and Sauteed Mushrooms for dinner

# Day 3

**Breakfast:** Granola with Greek yoghourt and honey for breakfast

**Lunch:** Chickpea and lentil soup for lunch.

**Dinner:** Mango Tofu Pie with Brown Rice for dinner.

# Day 4

**Breakfast:** blueberry muffins


*Complete Acid-Reflux Cookbook for Beginners*

**Lunch:** Chicken and barley stew for lunch

**Dinner:** serve baked french fries and black bean burgers.

## Day 5

**Breakfast:** Turkey White Bean Soup

**Lunch:** French Toast with Cinnamon.

**Dinner:** Chickpea salad with seared salmon for dinner

## Day 6

**Breakfast:** Roasted vegetable breakfast tacos.

**Lunch:** lentil and chickpea soup

**Dinner:** Spring Vegetable Quinoa Salad for dinner

## Day 7

**Breakfast:** Sweet potato toast with ginger honey.

**Lunch:** Chicken and black-eyed pea soup for lunch

**Dinner:** Udon Noodle Salad with Salmon for dinner

# Week 2

## Day 8

**Breakfast:** Green Smoothie with Spinach and Mixed Berries.

**Lunch:** Stuffed Mushrooms with Tomato and Basil

**Dinner:** Roasted vegetables and chicken with basil pesto

## Day 9

**Breakfast:** Chia seed pudding with fresh fruit.

**Lunch:** Lentil burgers with slices of avocado.


*Complete Acid-Reflux Cookbook
for Beginners*

**Dinner:** Quinoa and asparagus with grilled shrimp on skewers.

## Day 10

**Breakfast:** Almond butter and banana toast

**Lunch:** bok choy slaw and grilled chicken.

**Dinner:** Quinoa- and black-bean-stuffed bell peppers

## Day 11

**Breakfast:** Raspberry Coconut Chia Pudding

**Lunch:** Tuna salad lettuce wraps


*Complete Acid-Reflux Cookbook for Beginners*

**Dinner:** Baked cod with lemon-garlic green beans.

## Day 12

**Breakfast:** Parsnip French fries with Garlic Aioli

**Lunch:** Avocado and tomato omelette

**Dinner:** Chickpea salad with feta cheese from the Mediterranean

## Day 13

**Breakfast:** Acai bowl with fresh fruit toppings.

**Lunch:** Homemade Caesar Salad with Chicken

**Dinner:** Grilled sirloin steak and roasted Brussels sprouts

## Day 14

**Breakfast:** Sweet potato hash with poached eggs.

**Lunch:** Cucumber and red onion in a Greek quinoa salad

**Dinner:** Quinoa and asparagus with baked salmon.

# Week 3

## Day 15

**Breakfast:** Mixed berry smoothie bowl

**Lunch:** spinach and feta-stuffed chicken breast.

**Dinner:** Vegetarian Stuffed Bell Peppers

## Day 16

**Breakfast:** Caprese salad with balsamic glaze

**Lunch:** Veggie omelet.

**Dinner:** Grilled vegetable skewers with tofu

## Day 17

**Breakfast:** Papaya and Lime Smoothie

**Lunch:** Quinoa and black bean salad

**Dinner:** Grilled chicken with lemon and herbs and cauliflower rice.

## Day 18

**Breakfast:** Coconut chia pudding with mango slices.

**Lunch:** Greek chickpea salad with red wine vinaigrette for lunch.

**Dinner:** Teriyaki salmon and sautéed spinach.

## Day 19

**Breakfast:** Mixed Fruit Salad with Honey-Lime Dressing

**Lunch:** Stuffed Portobello Mushrooms with Quinoa

**Dinner:** Grilled zucchini and squash with pesto

## Day 20

**Breakfast:** A Green Tea Smoothie.

**Lunch:** Lentil Salad with Roasted Vegetables

**Dinner:** Green beans and herb-roasted turkey breast

## Day 21

**Breakfast:** Greek yoghourt parfait with berries and almonds

**Lunch:** Chickpea and Roasted Vegetable Salad

**Dinner:** Lemon Garlic Shrimp and Cauliflower Mash.

# Chapter Three

## Breakfast

### Banana-walnut Muffins.

**Ingredients:**

- One cup of all-purpose flour
- One cup of whole wheat flour
- One teaspoon of baking powder.
- 0.5 teaspoon baking soda
- 1/2 cup of melted unsalted butter
- 1/4 teaspoon of salt
- Brown sugar, 3/4 cup
- 2 big, mashed, ripe bananas
- 2 eggs, big

- 1/2 cup finely chopped walnuts
- 1 teaspoon vanilla essence

## Instructions:

1. Line a muffin pan with paper liners and preheat your oven to 350°F (175°C).
2. Combine the flour, baking powder, baking soda, and salt in a large basin.
3. Combine the melted butter, brown sugar, eggs, vanilla extract, and mashed bananas in a separate dish.
4. Stirring constantly, add the wet components to the dry ingredients gradually.


*Complete Acid-Reflux Cookbook for Beginners*

5. Gently include the walnut halves.

6. Evenly distribute the batter among the muffin tins.

7. Bake the muffins for 18 to 20 minutes, or until a toothpick inserted in the middle comes out clean.

8. After the muffins have cooled in the pan for a few minutes, move them to a wire rack to finish cooling.

# Pancakes with Buttermilk

## Ingredients:

- 2 tablespoons granulated sugar
- 1 teaspoon baking powder
- 1 cup all-purpose flour.
- 0.5 teaspoon baking soda
- 1 cup buttermilk
- 1/4 teaspoon of salt
- One big egg
- 2 tablespoons of melted unsalted butter
- Cooking spray or more melted butter for the pan

## Instructions:

1. A large bowl should be used to mix the flour, sugar, baking soda, and salt.

2. Combine the buttermilk, egg, and melted butter in another bowl.

3. Combine the dry ingredients by adding the wet components and stirring just until incorporated. There should still be some lumps in the batter.

4. Lightly oil a nonstick pan or griddle with cooking spray or melted butter and heat over medium heat.


*Complete Acid-Reflux Cookbook
for Beginners*

5. For each pancake, pour 1/4 cup of the batter into the skillet.

6. Cook the pancake for two to three minutes, or until surface bubbles appear and the edges seem to be set.

7. After flipping the pancakes, fry them for a further 1-2 minutes, or until they are well cooked and golden brown.

8. Serve warm with your preferred garnishes, such as a dollop of Greek yoghourt, fresh fruit, or maple syrup.

# Grasshopper

## Ingredients:

- 2 cups old-fashioned oats
- 1/2 cup chopped nuts (walnuts, pecans, or almonds) are required.
- 1/4 cup coconut shreds without added sugar
- 2 tablespoons maple syrup or honey
- 2 tablespoons of melted coconut oil
- 1/4 tsp salt
- 1 teaspoon vanilla essence
- 1/2 cup dried fruit (apricots, raisins, or cranberries)

## Instructions:

1. A baking sheet should be lined with parchment paper and your oven should be preheated to 325°F (160°C).

2. Combine the oats, chopped almonds, and shredded coconut in a large bowl.

3. In another dish, combine the salt, vanilla essence, melted coconut oil, honey or maple syrup, and honey.

4. After adding the wet mixture to the dry ingredients, whisk everything together well.

5. Evenly distribute the granola on the lined baking sheet.



*Complete Acid-Reflux Cookbook for Beginners*

6. Bake for 15-20 minutes, stirring halfway through to achieve equal browning, or until the granola is golden brown.

7. Before adding the dried fruits, let the granola cool fully on the baking pan.

8. You may keep the granola for up to two weeks in an airtight container. Take pleasure in milk, yoghourt, or as a garnish for smoothie bowls.

# Blueberry Muffins

## Ingredients:

- 1/2 cup granulated sugar
- 1 1/2 cups all-purpose flour
- 2 teaspoons baking powder
- 1/2 cup milk
- 1/4 tsp. salt
- 14 cups of vegetable oil
- One big egg, one teaspoon of vanilla essence, and one cup of fresh blueberries.

## Instructions:

- A muffin tray should be lined with paper liners and your oven


*Complete Acid-Reflux Cookbook
for Beginners*

should be preheated at 400°F (200°C).

- Combine the flour, sugar, baking soda, and salt in a large basin.

- In another dish, thoroughly blend the milk, vegetable oil, egg, and vanilla essence.

- Stirring constantly, add the wet components to the dry ingredients gradually.

- Carefully incorporate the fresh blueberries.

- Evenly distribute the batter among the muffin tins.

- Bake the muffins for 15 to 18 minutes, or until a toothpick


*Complete Acid-Reflux Cookbook for Beginners*

inserted in the middle comes out clean.

- After the muffins have cooled in the pan for a few minutes, move them to a wire rack to finish cooling.

## French Toast

### Ingredients:

- 2 big eggs
- 4 pieces of bread, either white, whole wheat or multigrain.
- A cup of milk
- 1/4 teaspoon powdered cinnamon
- 1 teaspoon vanilla extract

**Instructions:**

- For the skillet, use butter or frying spray. For the dish, use maple syrup and fresh berries.

- A small dish should be used to whisk the eggs, milk, vanilla essence, and ground cinnamon.

- Place a nonstick griddle or skillet over medium heat and cover the bottom with a thin layer of cooking spray or butter.

- Coat both sides of each piece of bread well by dipping it into the egg mixture.

- Add the bread pieces to the pan and cook for 2 to 3 minutes on each side, or until golden and thoroughly heated through.

- Plate the warm French toast and top it with fresh berries and maple syrup.

## Breakfast Tacos Made with Roasted Vegetables

### Ingredients:

- A small sweet potato that has been peeled and chopped
- A red bell pepper that has been cut.
- 1 thinly sliced tiny zucchini
- 1 tablespoon olive oil

- 4 small whole wheat or corn tortillas
- Salt and pepper to taste
- 4 eggs, big
- Slices of avocado and salsa for serving

## Instructions:

1. A baking sheet should be lined with parchment paper and your oven should be preheated to 400°F (200°C).

2. Combine olive oil, salt, and pepper with the chopped sweet potato, red bell pepper, and zucchini.

3. Arrange the veggies on the prepared baking sheet in a single layer.

4. Roast the veggies in the oven for 20 to 25 minutes, stirring halfway through, or until they are soft and slightly caramelised.

5. Warm the tortillas for one minute on each side in a dry skillet over medium heat while the veggies roast.

6. Cook the eggs in the same skillet to your preferred level of doneness (fried, scrambled, or sunny-side-up).

7. To make the morning tacos, spread some of the roasted veggies and scrambled eggs onto each tortilla.

8. Place avocado slices and salsa on top before folding the tortillas to make tacos. Serve right away.

## Sweet Potato Toast with Honey and Ginger

**Ingredients:**

- 1 big sweet potato, rinsed and cut into 1/4-inch-thick slices down the length

- 2 tablespoons softened unsalted butter
- 1 tablespoon honey
- 1/2 teaspoon ginger root
- A dash of salt
- Suggestions for toppings include toasted coconut flakes, almond butter, and banana slices.

## Instructions:

1. A baking sheet should be lined with parchment paper and your oven should be preheated to 400°F (200°C).

2. Arrange the slices of sweet potato on the lined baking sheet.


*Complete Acid-Reflux Cookbook
for Beginners*

3. Combine the softened butter, honey, ground ginger, and salt in a small bowl.

4. Apply a layer of ginger-honey butter to each slice of sweet potato.

5. Bake sweet potatoes in the oven for 15 to 20 minutes, or until they are soft and slightly caramelised.

6. Let your preferred garnishes, such as almond butter, sliced bananas, and toasty coconut flakes, sit on top of the sweet potato slices while they are still somewhat warm.

# Chapter Four

## Soups and Stews

## Chicken Noodle Soup

### Ingredients:

- 1 tablespoon olive oil
- 2 medium carrots
- 2 celery stalks
- 1 medium onion, diced
- 2 minced garlic cloves.
- 2 cups of cooked, shredded chicken
- 6 cups of chicken broth
- 1 bay leaf

- 1/2 tsp dried thyme
- Salt & pepper to taste
- Fresh parsley for decoration
- 1 cup egg noodles or pasta of your choice

## Instructions:

1. The olive oil should be heated over medium heat in a big saucepan or Dutch oven.

2. Include the diced celery, carrots, and onion and sauté for 5 to 6 minutes, or until the veggies are tender.

3. Add the garlic powder and simmer for an additional one to two minutes.

4. Add the egg noodles, bay leaf, and dried thyme after adding the chicken stock and shredded chicken.

5. After the soup comes to a boil, lower the heat to a simmer and cook the noodles for 10 to 12 minutes.

6. Taste-testingly season with salt and pepper.

7. Before serving, remove the bay leaf.

8. Top with fresh parsley and serve immediately.

# Eggplant Soup

## Ingredients:

- 2 huge eggplants, diced after being skinned
- 1 large onion
- 2 cloves minced garlic.
- 2 tablespoons olive oil
- 1 can (14 oz) chopped tomatoes, with juice
- 4 cups vegetable broth
- 1/8 teaspoon dried oregano
- 1/2 teaspoon dried basil
- Salt and pepper to taste
- Garnish with fresh basil leaves

## Instructions:

1. The olive oil should be heated over medium heat in a big saucepan or Dutch oven.

2. Stir in the minced garlic and onion, and cook for an additional 5–6 minutes, or until the onion is transparent.

3. Include the chopped eggplant and continue cooking for an additional 5 to 6 minutes, or until the eggplant begins to soften.

4. Add the vegetable broth, the diced tomatoes, and their juice, along with the dried oregano and basil.



*Complete Acid-Reflux Cookbook
for Beginners*

5. After the soup comes to a boil, lower the heat to a simmer and cook the soup for 20 to 25 minutes, or until the eggplant is fork-tender.

6. Puree the soup using an immersion blender until it is smooth. The soup may also be added to a blender and blended in batches.

7. To taste, add salt and pepper to the food.

8. Before serving, garnish with fresh basil leaves.

# Chicken and Kellogg's Stew

## Ingredients:

- 1 tbsp olive oil
- 1 lb of diced, skinless, boneless chicken breasts.
- 1 sliced medium onion
- 2 sliced and peeled carrots
- 2 cut celery stalks
- 2 minced garlic cloves
- 1 cup pearl barley
- 6 cups chicken broth
- 1 bay leaf,
- 1/2 tsp. dried thyme, salt, and pepper to taste
- Garnish with fresh parsley


*Complete Acid-Reflux Cookbook for Beginners*

## Instructions:

1. The olive oil should be heated over medium heat in a big saucepan or Dutch oven.

2. Include the diced celery, carrots, and onion and sauté for 5 to 6 minutes, or until the veggies are tender.

3. Continue cooking for an additional 1–2 minutes after adding the minced garlic.

4. Include the bite-sized chicken pieces and sauté them until they are just beginning to brown.

5. Pour the chicken stock over the pearl barley, add the bay leaf, and stir in the dried thyme.


*Complete Acid-Reflux Cookbook
for Beginners*

6. The stew should be brought to a boil, then simmer for 30 to 35 minutes, or until the barley is soft and the chicken is well cooked.

7. To taste, add salt and pepper to the food.

8. Before serving, remove the bay leaf.

9. Top with fresh parsley and serve immediately.



*Complete Acid-Reflux Cookbook for Beginners*

# Black-Eyed Pea and Chicken Soup

## Ingredients:

- 1 tablespoon olive oil
- 2 medium carrots
- 2 celery stalks
- 1 medium onion, diced
- 2 minced garlic cloves.
- 2 cups of cooked
- Shredded chicken and 6 cups of chicken broth
- 1 can (15 oz) washed and drained black-eyed peas
- 1 bay leaf
- 1/2 tsp. dried thyme, salt, and pepper to taste


*Complete Acid-Reflux Cookbook
for Beginners*

- Garnish with fresh parsley

## Instructions:

1. The olive oil should be heated over medium heat in a big saucepan or Dutch oven.
2. Include the diced celery, carrots, and onion and sauté for 5 to 6 minutes, or until the veggies are tender.
3. Add the garlic powder and simmer for an additional one to two minutes.
4. Add the shredded chicken, black-eyed peas, bay leaf, and dried thyme after pouring in the chicken broth.


*Complete Acid-Reflux Cookbook for Beginners*

5. After the soup comes to a boil, turn the heat down to low and let it simmer for 10 to 12 minutes, depending on how well the flavours have combined.

6. Taste-testingly season with salt and pepper.

7. Before serving, remove the bay leaf.

8. Top with fresh parsley and serve immediately.

## Soup with Chickpeas and Lentils

**Ingredients:**

- 2 tbsp olive oil, 1 big onion

- 2 peeled and diced carrots
- 2 celery stalks.
- 2 minced garlic cloves
- 1 cup washed and drained dry lentils
- One can of chopped tomatoes with juice (14 ounces).
- 6 cups vegetarian broth
- One (15 oz) container of rinsed and drained chickpeas
- 1/2 tsp ground coriander
- 1 tsp ground cumin
- Season with salt and pepper to taste
- Garnish with fresh cilantro


*Complete Acid-Reflux Cookbook
for Beginners*

## Instructions:

1. The olive oil should be heated over medium heat in a big saucepan or Dutch oven.

2. Stir in the chopped celery, onion, and carrots, and cook for an additional 5 to 6 minutes, or until the veggies are tender.

3. Add the garlic powder and simmer for an additional one to two minutes.

4. Combine the chickpeas, ground cumin, and ground coriander with the dry lentils, diced tomatoes (and their juice), vegetable broth, and dried lentils.


*Complete Acid-Reflux Cookbook
for Beginners*

5. After bringing the soup to a boil, lower the heat to a simmer and cook the lentils for 20 to 25 minutes, depending on how soft you want your lentils.

6. Taste-testingly season with salt and pepper.

7. Before serving, garnish with fresh cilantro.

## Turkey White Bean Soup

### Ingredients:

- One tablespoon of olive oil
- one pound of ground turkey
- One medium onion diced
- two carrots peeled and cut

- Two celery stalks sliced

- 2 minced garlic cloves

- 2 cans (15 oz each) of chicken or turkey broth

- 6 cups total. drained and washed white beans

- 1 bay leaf

- 1/2 tsp. dried thyme, salt, and pepper to taste

- Garnish with fresh parsley

## Instructions:

- The olive oil should be heated over medium heat in a big saucepan or Dutch oven

- Include the diced celery, carrots, and onion and sauté for 5 to 6


*Complete Acid-Reflux Cookbook
for Beginners*

minutes, or until the veggies are tender.

- Add the garlic powder and simmer for an additional one to two minutes.

- Include the ground turkey and cook it through and until it is browned.

- Add the white beans, bay leaf, and dried thyme after adding the chicken or turkey stock.

- After bringing the soup to a boil, turn the heat down to low and let it simmer for 15 to 20 minutes to let the flavours blend.

- To taste, add salt and pepper to the food
- Before serving, remove the bay leaf.
- Top with fresh parsley and serve immediately.
- Enjoy the cosiness of stews and soups.


*Complete Acid-Reflux Cookbook for Beginners*

# Chapter Five

## Sides and Snacks

## Low-Acid Tomato Sauce

### Ingredients:

- 1 (14 oz) can of crushed tomatoes
- 2 minced garlic cloves
- 1 teaspoon dried oregano
- 1 tablespoon olive oil
- One tablespoon of dried basil
- To taste, salt and pepper

## Instructions:

1. Heat the olive oil in a saucepan over medium heat. Sauté the minced garlic until fragrant after adding it.

2. Add salt, pepper, dried oregano, dry basil, and smashed tomatoes.

3. Simmer the sauce for 15 to 20 minutes over low heat, stirring regularly.

4. Take it off the stove and allow it to cool before using it as a sauce or dip for your preferred foods.


*Complete Acid-Reflux Cookbook for Beginners*

# Basil Pesto

## Ingredients:

- 2 cups packed fresh basil leaves
- Half a cup of grated Parmesan cheese
- Half a cup of pine nuts or walnuts
- 3 minced garlic cloves
- Half a cup of olive oil
- To taste, salt and pepper

## Instructions:

1. Place the basil, Parmesan cheese, pine nuts or walnuts, and minced garlic in a food processor.

2. Slowly add the olive oil while the food processor is running until the mixture is creamy and smooth.
3. To taste, add salt and pepper to the dish.
4. Apply the pesto to pasta and other foods as a sauce, spread, or dip.

## Mashed Potatoes with Ginger

**Ingredients:**
- 2 pounds of chunked, peeled russet potatoes

- 1 tablespoon freshly grated ginger
- 1/4 cup unsalted butter
- 1/4 cup milk
- To taste, salt and pepper

## Instructions:

1. In a big saucepan of salted water, boil the potato pieces until they are soft. Drain again and add to the pot.

2. Melt the butter in a small saucepan over low heat. Grated ginger is added and cooked for a couple of minutes until aromatic.


*Complete Acid-Reflux Cookbook for Beginners*

3. Add the milk and butter with the ginger to the potatoes, then mash until smooth and creamy.

4. To taste, add salt and pepper to the dish. Use it as a hearty side dish.

# French Fries that are Baked

## Ingredients:

- Four huge russet potatoes, thinly sliced
- 1 teaspoon paprika
- 2 tablespoons olive oil
- Half a teaspoon of garlic powder
- To taste, salt and pepper


*Complete Acid-Reflux Cookbook for Beginners*

## Instructions:

1. Set the oven temperature to 450°F (230°C). Use parchment paper to cover a baking sheet.
2. Combine the potato strips with olive oil, paprika, garlic powder, salt, and pepper in a large basin.
3. Arrange the seasoned potatoes on the preheated baking sheet in a single layer.
4. Bake the fries in a preheated oven for 25 to 30 minutes, or until they are crisp and golden. Enjoy without feeling guilty!



*Complete Acid-Reflux Cookbook for Beginners*

# Bok Choy Slaw

## Ingredients:

- 2 teaspoons rice vinegar
- 4 cups thinly sliced bok choy
- 1 cup shredded carrots
- 1/4 cup chopped green onions
- 1 tablespoon low-sodium soy sauce
- 1 tablespoon maple syrup or honey
- 1 tsp. toasted sesame oil
- Sesame seeds as an optional garnish

## Instructions:

- Combine the sliced bok choy, shredded carrots, and finely chopped green onions in a big bowl.

- Combine the low-sodium soy sauce, honey, maple syrup, and toasted sesame oil in a separate small bowl.

- After adding the dressing, blend the bok choy mixture thoroughly.

- If desired, add sesame seeds as a garnish. Serve as a crisp and energising side salad.

# French Fries with Parsnips

## Ingredients:

- 4 big parsnips that have been peeled and thinly sliced
- 1 teaspoon paprika
- 2 tablespoons olive oil
- Half a teaspoon of garlic powder
- To taste, salt and pepper

## Instructions:

1. Set the oven temperature to 425°F (220°C). Use parchment paper to cover a baking sheet.
2. Combine the parsnip strips with the olive oil, paprika, garlic

powder, salt, and pepper in a large bowl.

3. Place the seasoned parsnips on the preheated baking sheet in a single layer.

4. Bake the parsnips in the preheated oven for 20 to 25 minutes, or until they are crispy and just beginning to colour.

## Stuffed Mushroom Caps

### Ingredients:

- 12 big mushroom caps, stems cut off
- 1/2 cup melted cream cheese
- 2 minced garlic cloves


*Complete Acid-Reflux Cookbook for Beginners*

- 1/4 cup grated Parmesan cheese
- 1/4 cup chopped fresh parsley
- To taste, salt and pepper

## Instructions:

- Preheat the oven temperature is set at 375°F (190°C). Use parchment paper to cover a baking sheet.

- Combine the cream cheese, grated Parmesan cheese, parsley, minced garlic, salt, and pepper in a medium bowl.

- After stuffing the cream cheese mixture into each mushroom cap, arrange them on the prepared baking sheet.

- Bake for 15 to 20 minutes, or until the filling is brown and the mushrooms are soft, in the preheated oven.

# Chapter Six

## Salads

### Salad with Asparagus and Green Beans

**Ingredients:**

- 1 bunch of asparagus, chopped into bite-sized pieces after trimming.
- 1 cup green beans, trimmed and cut in half
- 1/4 cup toasted sliced almonds
- Lemon juice, 2 teaspoons
- Two tablespoons of extra virgin olive oil

- One teaspoon of Dijon mustard, and salt & pepper to taste

## Instructions:

1. Blanch the asparagus and green beans in a saucepan of boiling water for two to three minutes, or until they are crisp-tender. To end cooking, drain and rinse with cold water.

2. To create the dressing, combine the lemon juice, olive oil, Dijon mustard, salt, and pepper in a small bowl.

3. Place the green beans and asparagus that have been blanched in a serving dish. Over

the veggies, drizzle the dressing and toss to coat.

4. To add crunch and nutty taste, sprinkle roasted, thinly sliced almonds on top of the salad.

## Blue Cheese Dressed with Iceberg Wedge Salad

**Ingredients:**

- One small head of cut-up iceberg lettuce
- 1/4 cup blue cheese crumbles
- 1/4 cup Greek yoghourt without added sugar
- Mayonnaise, 2 tablespoons

- Two tablespoons of freshly chopped white wine vinegar and chives.
- To taste, salt and pepper

## Instructions:

- Position the wedges of iceberg lettuce on a serving plate.
- To create the dressing, mix the crumbled blue cheese, mayonnaise, white wine vinegar, chopped chives, salt, and pepper in a small basin.
- Dress the lettuce wedges with the blue cheese dressing.


*Complete Acid-Reflux Cookbook
for Beginners*

- For any occasion, serve the salad as a light appetiser or side dish.

# Chinese Chicken Salad

## Ingredients:

- 2 cups of cooked chicken breast that has been shredded
- 2 cups of Napa cabbage
- 1 cup of carrots
- 1/4 cup of green onions.
- 2 teaspoons soy sauce
- 1/4 cup toasted almond slices
- 1 teaspoon grated fresh ginger
- 2 tablespoons rice vinegar
- 1 tablespoon sesame oil

- 1 tablespoon honey or maple syrup
- Sesame seeds for decoration (optional)

## Instructions:

- Combine the shredded chicken breast, shredded carrots, chopped green onions, Napa cabbage, and toasted sliced almonds in a big bowl.
- To create the dressing, combine the soy sauce, rice vinegar, sesame oil, honey, or maple syrup, and freshly grated ginger in a separate small bowl.

- After adding the dressing, toss the chicken and vegetable mixture to thoroughly coat.

- If desired, add sesame seeds as a garnish. Serve as a healthy and filling alternative for lunch or supper.

## Salmon and Udon Noodle Salad

### Ingredients:

- 8 ounces of cooked udon noodles by the directions on the package

- 1/2 cup cooked and shelled edamame beans

- 1 cup thinly sliced cucumber
- 1 cup flaked cooked salmon
- 1/4 cup sliced green onions
- 2 teaspoons soy sauce
- 1 teaspoon of honey or maple syrup
- 1 tablespoon of sesame oil
- Sesame seeds for garnish (optional)

## Instructions:

1. Place the cooked udon noodles, flaked salmon, thinly sliced cucumber, cooked edamame beans, and thinly sliced green onions in a large bowl.

2. To create the dressing, combine the soy sauce, sesame oil, rice vinegar, honey, or maple syrup in a separate small bowl.

3. Add the dressing to the bowl of noodles and salmon, then toss to incorporate.

4. If desired, add sesame seeds as a garnish. Serve the salmon and udon noodle salad as a filling and delicious lunch or supper alternative.

# Salad Made with Seared Salmon and Chickpeas

## Ingredients:

- 2 salmon fillets
- 1 can (15 oz) washed and drained chickpeas
- 1 cup halved cherry tomatoes
- 1/4 cup red onion and fresh parsley minced
- 2 tablespoons lemon juice
- 1 teaspoon of ground cumin
- 2 tablespoons of extra virgin olive oil, and salt & pepper to taste

## Instructions:

- Sprinkle salt, pepper, and ground cumin over the salmon fillets.

- Heat 1 tablespoon of olive oil in a pan over medium-high heat. Add the salmon fillets and heat until fully cooked for 3–4 minutes on each side.

- Combine the chickpeas, cherry tomatoes, red onion, and fresh parsley in a big bowl.

- To prepare the dressing, combine the lemon juice, remaining olive oil, salt, and pepper in a separate small dish.


*Complete Acid-Reflux Cookbook
for Beginners*

- After adding the dressing, mix the chickpea salad well.
- Place the seared salmon fillets on top of the salad. Use as a filling and substantial supper choice.

## Spring Vegetable Quinoa Salad

**Ingredients:**

- One cup of cooked quinoa
- One cup of chopped blanched asparagus
- One cup of blanched green peas
- One cup of diced radishes.
- 14 cups finely minced fresh mint

- 1/4 cup feta cheese that has been crumbled
- 2 teaspoons lemon juice
- 1 tablespoon honey or maple syrup
- 2 tablespoons olive oil
- To taste, salt and pepper

## Instructions:

1. Combine the cooked quinoa, diced radishes, blanched green peas, chopped fresh mint, and feta cheese in a large bowl.

2. To create the dressing, combine the lemon juice, olive oil, honey (or maple syrup), salt, and pepper in a separate small bowl.


*Complete Acid-Reflux Cookbook
for Beginners*

3. Drizzle the dressing over the quinoa and vegetable combination, then toss to evenly distribute the dressing.

4. Offer the spring vegetable quinoa salad as a healthy vegetarian lunch alternative or as a light and refreshing side dish.


*Complete Acid-Reflux Cookbook
for Beginners*

# Chapter Seven

## Main Courses

### Cashew Chicken

**Ingredients:**

- A pound of boneless Skinless chicken breasts that have been diced into bite-sized portions
- One-fourth cup of low-sodium soy sauce
- 2 teaspoons of oyster sauce
- Hoisin sauce, 2 teaspoons
- 2 chopped garlic cloves
- 1 teaspoon grated fresh ginger

- 1 tablespoon rice vinegar
- 1 tablespoon honey
- 1/2 cup cashews, unsalted
- 2 chopped green onions
- 1 tablespoon of vegetable oil
- Brown rice cooked and ready to serve.

## Instructions:

1. Soy sauce, oyster sauce, hoisin sauce, rice vinegar, honey, garlic, and ginger should all be combined in a bowl. Mix thoroughly.

2. Using a large pan over medium-high heat, warm the vegetable oil. Add the chicken

and heat it through until it is browned.

3. When the chicken is properly coated, pour the sauce mixture over it. Cook the cashews and green onions for a further two to three minutes.

4. Overcooked brown rice, please.

# Chicken with Mushrooms in a Sauté

**Ingredients:**

- 1 pound of skinless, boneless chicken thighs or breasts
- 8 ounces of cut cremini mushrooms

- 1 tablespoon of olive oil
- 2 minced garlic cloves
- 1/4 cup heavy cream
- 1/2 cup chicken broth
- 1 tablespoon of thyme leaves, fresh
- To serve, cooked quinoa or wild rice with salt and pepper to taste

## Instructions:

- Salt and pepper the chicken before cooking it. Olive oil should be heated to a medium-high haze in a big skillet. Add the chicken and heat it through, browning it on both sides. Take out of the skillet and put aside

- Sliced mushrooms should be added to the same pan and cooked until they release moisture and become golden brown. Cook for one more minute before adding the minced garlic.

- Scrape any browned pieces from the bottom of the pan, then pour in the chicken broth. Simmer for a while.

- Add fresh thyme leaves and heavy cream after mixing. Add salt and pepper to taste.


*Complete Acid-Reflux Cookbook for Beginners*

- Then add the cooked chicken back to the skillet and boil the mixture for a few minutes.
- Serve with cooked wild rice or quinoa.

## Mango Tofu Opia

### Ingredients:

- Cubed one block of firm tofu
- Two teaspoons of cornstarch
- Two tablespoons of vegetable oil are the ingredients.
- 2 chopped green onions
- 1/2 cup sliced ripe mango
- 1/4 cup diced red bell pepper
- 2 teaspoons soy sauce

- 1 teaspoon sesame oil

- 1 teaspoon rice vinegar

- 1 tablespoon of honey.

- Prepared jasmine rice, to be served

## Instructions:

1. Follow these steps to cover the tofu cubes with cornstarch equally. Clear away any extra cornstarch.

2. Vegetable oil should be warmed up over medium-high heat in a big pan. Add the tofu and heat it until it is all crispy and golden brown. Take out of the skillet and put aside.

3. Include diced mango, red bell pepper, and green onions in the same pan. Cook until somewhat softened for 1-2 minutes.

4. Soy sauce, honey, rice vinegar, and sesame oil should all be combined in a small bowl. Mix the mango mixture with the sauce after pouring it over it.

5. Re-add the cooked tofu to the pan and toss it in the sauce gently.

6. Overcooked jasmine rice, please.


*Complete Acid-Reflux Cookbook for Beginners*

# Legumes Burgers

## Ingredients:

- 1 cup cooked lentils
- 1/2 cup rolled oats
- 1/2 cup carrots that have been shredded.
- 14 cups minced red onion
- 2 cloves minced garlic
- 1 teaspoon smoky paprika
- 1 teaspoon cumin - 1 tablespoon tomato paste
- Half a teaspoon of chilli powder
- To taste-adapted salt and pepper
- 2 tablespoons olive oil


*Complete Acid-Reflux Cookbook for Beginners*

- Whole grain buns for pairing with hamburgers
- Slices of lettuce, tomatoes, and avocado as toppings

## Instructions:

- Prepared lentils, rolled oats, grated carrots, red onion, garlic, tomato paste, cumin, smoked paprika, chilli powder, salt, and pepper should all be mixed in a food processor.
- Create hamburger patties out of the mixture. For 30 minutes, place them in the refrigerator to firm up on a tray covered with parchment paper.

- Olive oil should be heated in a big pan over medium heat. The lentil burgers should be roasted through and golden brown after 4-5 minutes on each side.

- Serve with lettuce, tomato slices, and slices of avocado on whole grain hamburger buns.

## Black Bean Burgers

**Ingredients:**

- 1 can (15 oz) drained and rinsed black beans
- 1/2 cup cooked quinoa
- /4 cup finely chopped red onion
- 2 minced garlic cloves.


*Complete Acid-Reflux Cookbook
for Beginners*

- 1 teaspoon each of cumin and chilli powder
- A half teaspoon of paprika
- Fresh cilantro, 1/4 cup minced
- Soy sauce, 1 tablespoon
- Olive oil, 1 tbsp
- Whole-wheat hamburger
- Buns for serving
- Lettuce, sliced red onion
- Sliced avocado for toppings

## Instructions:

1. Black beans should be mashed with a fork or potato masher in a large basin until nearly smooth.

2. Combine cooked quinoa with chopped red onion, minced garlic, soy sauce, ground cumin, chilli powder, paprika, and ground cumin. Combine well after mixing.

3. Create hamburger patties out of the mixture. For 30 minutes, place them in the refrigerator to firm up on a tray covered with parchment paper.

4. Olive oil is heated in a pan at medium temperature. The black bean burgers should be roasted through and crispy after 4-5 minutes on each side.

5. Serve with lettuce, sliced red onion, sliced avocado, and whole grain hamburger buns.

# Chicken with Red Potatoes

## Ingredients:

- Four skin-on, bone-in chicken thighs
- 1 pound of quartered red potatoes
- 1 tablespoon of olive oil
- 2 teaspoons of dried thyme
- 2 teaspoons of dried rosemary
- Fresh parsley, chopped, as a garnish
- Salt and pepper, to taste

## Instructions:

1. The oven should be preheated at 400°F (200°C).

2. Salt, pepper, dried thyme, and dried rosemary are used to season chicken thighs.

3. Olive oil should be heated over medium-high heat in a large oven-safe pan.

4. Cook the chicken thighs until the skin is brown and crispy by adding them with the skin side down. Cook for a further two minutes after flipping the chicken.

5. Red potatoes cut into quarters should be added to the pan and

mixed with the chicken's juices and oil.

6. When the chicken is cooked through and the potatoes are soft, place the skillet in the preheated oven and bake for 25 to 30 minutes.

7. Before serving, garnish with freshly cut parsley.

# Chapter Eight

## Desserts

## Healthy Apple Crisp

### Ingredients:

- 1 tablespoon lemon juice
- 4 medium-sized apples, peeled, cored, and thinly sliced.
- 1/4 cup almond flour
- 1/4 cup chopped almonds
- 1/2 cup rolled oats
- 2-tablespoons of maple syrup
- 1 teaspoon powdered cinnamon
- 1 tablespoon heated coconut oil

- Vanilla Greek yoghourt or low-fat ice cream, for serving
- A pinch of salt

## Instructions:

- The oven should be preheated at 375°F (190°C).

- Sliced apples should be placed in a baking dish after being mixed with lemon juice in a big basin.

- Rollin oats, almond flour, chopped almonds, maple syrup, melted coconut oil, ground cinnamon, and a dash of salt should all be combined in a separate bowl. Mix just enough to make the mixture crumbly.

- Over the apples in the baking dish, evenly distribute the oat mixture.

- Bake the topping for 25 to 30 minutes, or until golden brown and the apples are soft.

- Serve warm with low-fat ice cream or a dollop of vanilla Greek yoghourt.

# Vanilla Almond Pudding

## Ingredients:

- One cup of Greek yoghurt.
- 1/4 cup granola
- 1 teaspoon vanilla extract
- 2 tablespoons honey
- 1/4 cup chopped almonds
- Topping of fresh berries (strawberries, blueberries, and raspberries)

## Instructions:

1. Greek yoghourt, vanilla extract, and honey should all be well blended in a dish.

2. Layer the yoghourt mixture, granola, and sliced almonds in serving glasses or bowls, going up the glass until you reach the top.

3. Add fresh berries on top.

4. Serve right away or keep chilled until you're ready to.

## Rice Pudding with Coconut

**Ingredients:**

- 1 cup jasmine rice that hasn't been cooked
- 1 can (14 oz) coconut milk.
- Two cups of almond milk
- 1/4 cup maple syrup or honey


*Complete Acid-Reflux Cookbook
for Beginners*

- 1 teaspoon vanilla essence
- 1/8 teaspoon salt
- Flakes of toasty coconut, for garnish

## Instructions:

1. Uncooked jasmine rice, coconut milk, almond milk, honey or maple syrup, vanilla essence, and a dash of salt should all be combined in a pot.

2. Over medium-high heat, bring the mixture to a boil. Then, turn the heat down to low, cover the pan, and simmer for 20 to 25 minutes, or until the rice is done and the pudding has thickened.

3. To avoid sticking, stir every so while.

4. Take it off the fire and let it cool for a minute to cool.

5. Serve with toasted coconut flakes on top and warm or cold.

# Watermelon Pudding

## Ingredients:

- 1 cup Greek yoghourt
- 2 cups diced watermelon
- 1/4 cup granola
- 1 tablespoon honey
- Fresh mint leaves for decoration

## Instructions:

- Follow these steps to blend Greek yoghourt and honey into a dish.

- Layer cubed watermelon, yoghourt mixture, and granola in serving glasses or bowls, going up the sides of the glass each time.

- Add fresh mint leaves as a garnish.

- Serve right away.

# Honeydew Melon Chia Pudding

**Ingredients:**

- One-fourth cup of chia seeds
- One cup of unsweetened almond milk
- One tablespoon of honey
- Half a teaspoon of vanilla essence
- One cup of chopped honeydew melon.
- Fresh mint leaves for decoration

## Instructions:

1. Chia seeds, unsweetened almond milk, honey, and vanilla essence should all be well blended in a bowl

2. Allow the chia seeds to absorb the liquid and thicken into a pudding-like consistency by covering the bowl and placing it in the refrigerator for at least two hours or overnight.

3. Layer chia pudding and chopped honeydew melon in serving glasses or bowls, repeating the process until you reach the top of the glass.



*Complete Acid-Reflux Cookbook for Beginners*

4. Use fresh mint leaves as a garnish.

5. Offer cold.

## Banana and Blueberry Sorbet

**Ingredients:**

- 1 cup of frozen blueberries
- 2 ripe bananas, peeled and sliced.
- 1/2 cup unsweetened almond milk
- 1 tablespoon optional, taste-tested honey or maple syrup

- Slices of banana and fresh blueberries for topping

## Instructions:

- Place sliced bananas, frozen blueberries, unsweetened almond milk, and honey or maple syrup (if using) in a blender or food processor.
- When blending, add additional almond milk as necessary to get the desired consistency. Blend until smooth and creamy.
- Taste and, if necessary, adjust sweetness.
- Fill a container with the mixture, and place in the freezer


*Complete Acid-Reflux Cookbook
for Beginners*

for at least two hours, or until solid.

- Serve the sorbet in scoops with slices of banana and fresh blueberries on top.

# *Conclusion*

A big congratulations on finishing the "Complete Acid-Reflux Cookbook for Beginners."

You've learned important lessons about controlling acid reflux via a clean and pleasurable eating strategy.

You've made considerable progress in reducing discomfort and regaining balance in your life by comprehending how nutrition affects acid reflux symptoms and adhering to the 3-week meal plan.

Do not forget that this book is a guide to greater health and well-being rather than just a collection of recipes.

You now have the information and resources necessary to make wise decisions that support digestive harmony and lessen acid reflux symptoms.

The recipes offered here will satiate your palate while advancing your health objectives, whether you're looking for comforting breakfasts, invigorating lunches, beautiful dinners, or cool drinks.


*Complete Acid-Reflux Cookbook
for Beginners*

# Share the Power of Acid Reflux Relief with Others

We sincerely ask for your review if you found the "Complete Acid-Reflux Cookbook for Beginners" to be beneficial and transforming.

Your opinions and experiences will help others understand the advantages of this thorough guide.

Share your experience overcoming acid reflux and encourage other readers to adopt healthful, nutritious eating practices for better health.

Your review could influence someone's decision to adopt a better lifestyle and provide them with relief from acid reflux.

Your participation and comments are very helpful. To write a review and tell the world about your experience.

Let's keep moving forward toward better health one delicious and relaxing cuisine at a time!